7-Day Liver Detox Plan

Including Delicious Detoxifying Recipes

Table of Contents

Introduction

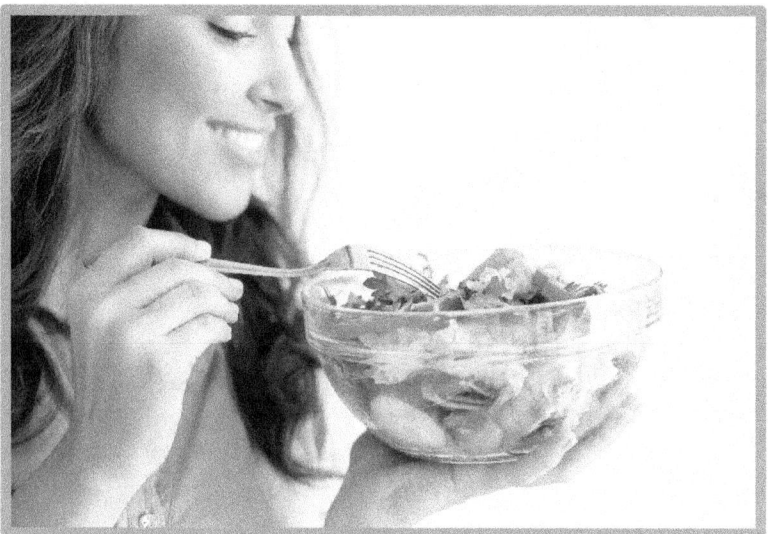

Each and every day you fill your body with toxins whether you know it or not. They can be found in the products you use, the food you eat and even the air you breathe. While your body has a natural detoxification system in place, if you put more toxins into your body than it can handle the excess will start to accumulate in your tissues and organs. Once your organs start to accumulate toxins they will be less effective and it could have devastating effects on your health. This is why a liver detox is so important – your liver is a vital organ and if it isn't functioning properly, your overall health will be impacted. In this book you will learn the basics about what a detox is and how it can benefit you. You will also receive tips for detoxing your liver as well as a collection of delicious detox recipes and a 7-day detox meal plan.

Chapter One: What is a Detox?

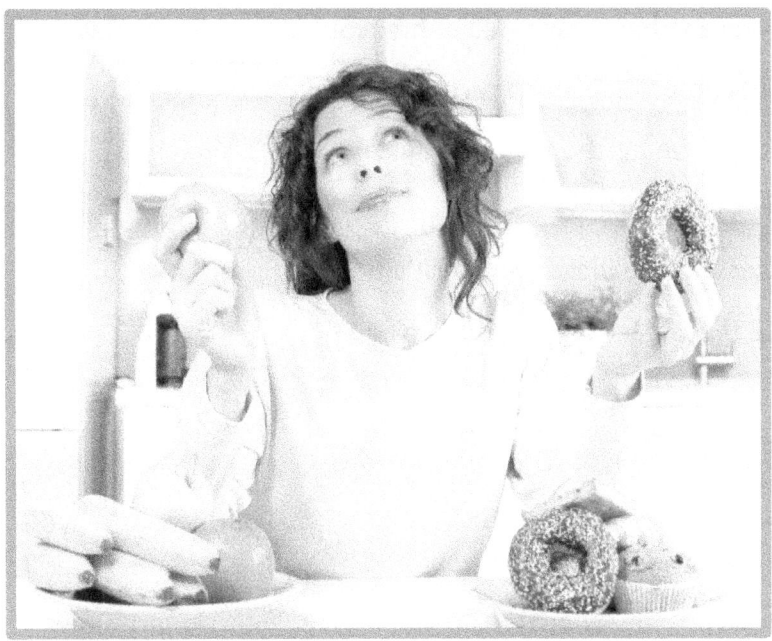

Before you can engage in a detox, you have to learn the basics about what a detox is. A detox is also sometimes referred to as a "cleanse" because that is what you are doing – you are cleansing your body of accumulated toxins in an effort to "reset" it, bringing it back to its intended function. In order to do this, you must remove the things from your life that are bringing toxins into your body. In many cases, those things are the food you eat. Processed foods, refined sugar/flour, fast food and other items are loaded with artificial ingredients, chemical preservatives and other substances which accumulate in your body and bring it into a state of toxicity. If you want to restore your body to full health, you need to remove those foods from your diet.

Benefits of a Detox

The main benefit of a liver detox is, of course, flushing excess toxins from your liver so it can return to its intended function. However, a detox has many other wide-reaching benefits for your body and your health as well. <u>Some other detox benefits include</u>:

- Increased energy levels, less fatigue

- Supports healthy weight loss by encouraging good eating habits
- Helps to support a healthy immune system
- Improved skin and hair health, fewer breakouts and stronger hair
- Reduced cravings for sugar and carbohydrates
- Improved cognitive function, clearer thinking, less brain fog
- Reduced breath odor
- Improved sense of wellbeing and positivity
- May reduce the impact of aging on skin and body

Chapter Two: How to Detox Your Liver

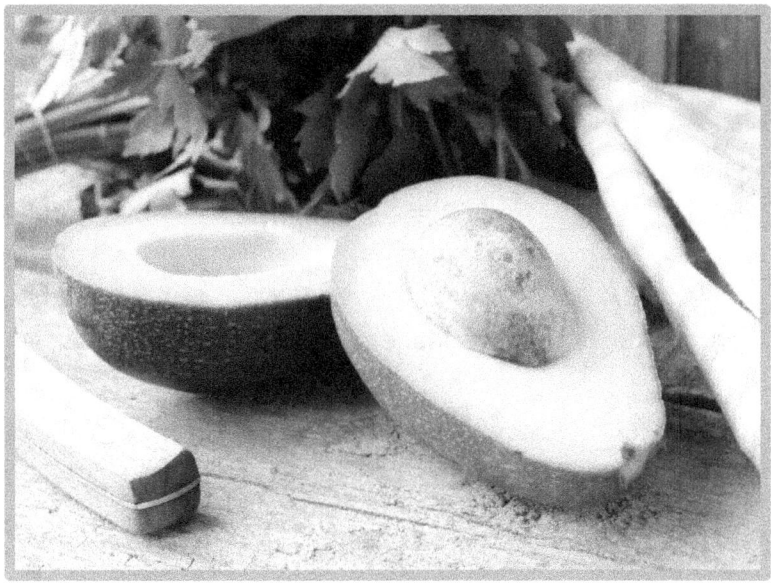

In order to detoxify your liver, and your body as a whole, you need to alter your eating habits. During your detox you should focus on healthy, wholesome foods rather than prepared and processed foods. Ideally, you should remove refined sugars and carbohydrates (this includes all-purpose flour and white/brown sugars) from your diet along with gluten-containing grains. Avoid artificial sweeteners, using only natural sweeteners like honey and maple syrup in moderation. Your diet should be founded on fresh produce and lean sources of protein like chicken and seafood, though you can feel free to enjoy beef, pork and game meat as well. During your 7-day detox it is wise to avoid soft drinks, alcoholic beverages and caffeine as well. In the next chapter you will receive a collection of healthy detox recipes to get you started.

Liver Detoxing Foods

When it comes to choosing the foods for your detox diet, it is essential that you stick to whole, natural foods. This means that you will have to exclude processed foods including refined sugars and flours from your diet as well as fast food, processed snacks and even soft drinks. In addition to removing these foods from your diet and focusing on natural foods, there are certain foods which have been shown to provide significant benefits specifically for detoxifying your liver. <u>Some of these foods include</u>:

- Brussels sprouts
- Garlic
- Dandelion greens
- Carrots
- Tomatoes
- Grapefruit
- Spinach
- Avocado
- Beets
- Asparagus
- Mustard greens
- Chicory
- Apples
- Quinoa
- Lemon
- Cabbage
- Lime
- Millet
- Turmeric
- Sesame seeds
- Ginger
- Fennel
- Flax seeds
- Parsley
- Artichoke

Chapter Three: Liver Detox Recipes

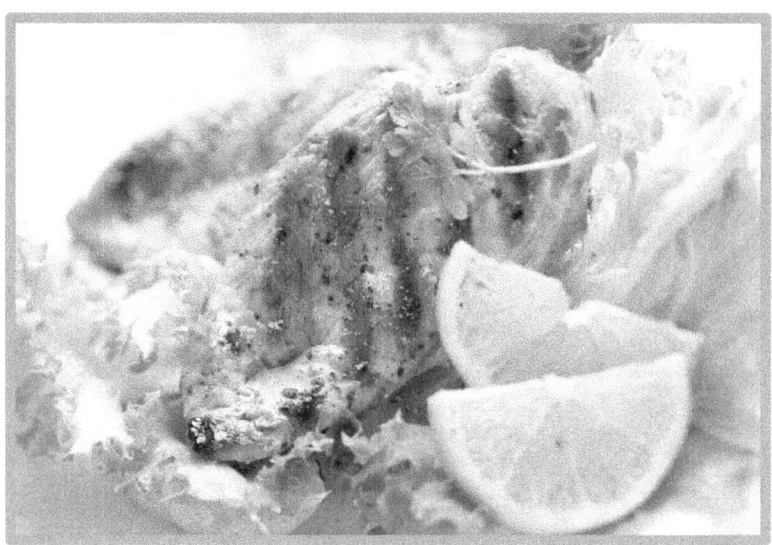

Recipes Included in this Book:

Banana Nut Muffins

Pumpkin Spice Pancakes

Tomato Zucchini Omelet

Blueberry Coconut Pancakes

Ham, Mushroom and Onion Frittata

Almond Flour Waffles

Veggie Egg White Omelet

Roasted Tomato Onion Soup

Walnut Apple Kale Salad

Chicken Apple Salad

Creamy Beet Soup

Red Cabbage Carrot Salad

Cream of Spinach Soup

Vegetable Quinoa Salad

Cilantro Herbed Turkey Burgers

Lemon Garlic Pork Tenderloin

Chipotle Lime Shrimp

Spicy Turkey Chili

Slow-Cooker Pulled Pork

Oven-Roasted Beef Tenderloin

Ginger Broccoli Stir-Fry

Lemon Pudding

Blueberry Crumble

Maple Pecan Cookies

Almond Flour Cupcakes

Strawberry Lime Sorbet

Baked Apples with Walnuts

Chocolate Coconut Cupcakes

Breakfast Recipes

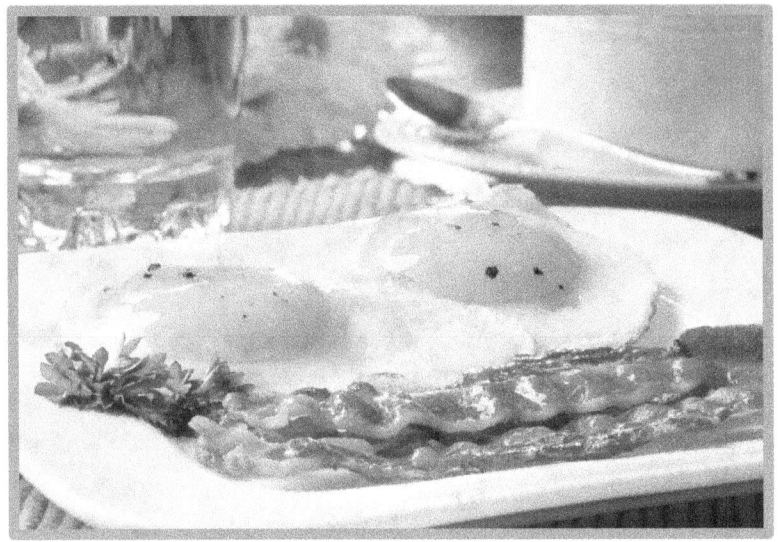

Recipes Included in this Section:

Banana Nut Muffins

Pumpkin Spice Pancakes

Tomato Zucchini Omelet

Blueberry Coconut Pancakes

Ham, Mushroom and Onion Frittata

Almond Flour Waffles

Veggie Egg White Omelet

Banana Nut Muffins

Servings: 12

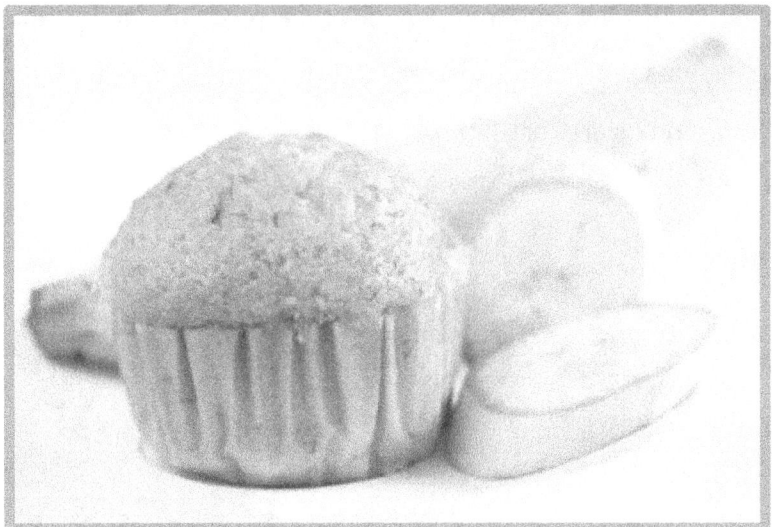

Ingredients:

- 3 tablespoons warm water
- 1 tablespoon chia seeds
- 1 cup buckwheat flour
- 1 teaspoon baking soda
- ¾ teaspoon ground cinnamon
- ¼ teaspoon ground nutmeg
- Pinch salt
- 1 ½ tablespoons coconut oil, melted
- 1 tablespoon cider vinegar
- 3 ripe bananas, mashed

Instructions:

1. Preheat the oven to 350°F and line a regular muffin pan with paper liners.
2. Whisk together the water and chia seeds in a small bowl and set aside for 5 minutes.
3. Combine the flour, baking soda, cinnamon, nutmeg and salt in a mixing bowl.
4. In a separate bowl, beat together the chia seed mixture, coconut oil and cider vinegar.

5. Whisk the dry ingredients into the wet until well combined then fold in the mashed banana and walnuts.

6. Spoon the batter into the prepared pan, filling each cup about 2/3 full.

7. Bake for 20 minutes until a knife inserted in the center of a muffin comes out clean.

8. Cool the muffins on a wire rack before serving.

Pumpkin Spice Pancakes

Servings: 4

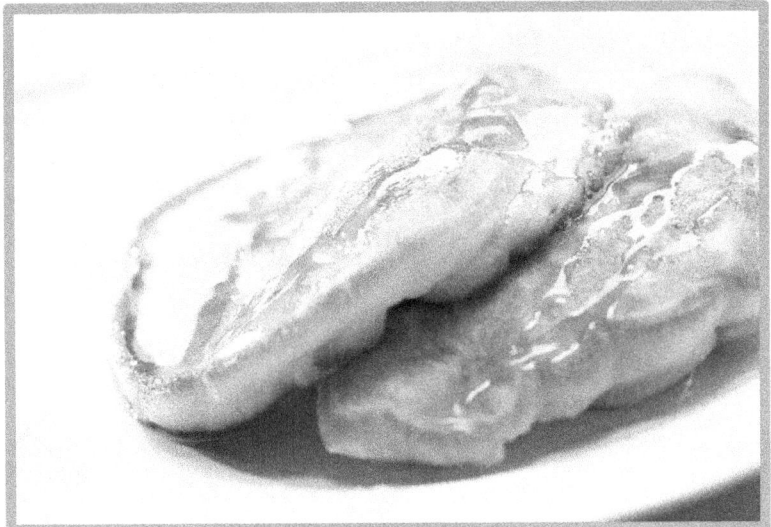

Ingredients:

- ¼ cup coconut flour
- 2 teaspoons ground cinnamon
- ¼ teaspoon baking soda
- Pinch salt
- 1 cup pumpkin puree
- 6 large eggs, lightly beaten

Instructions:

1. Combine the coconut flour, cinnamon, baking soda and salt in a mixing bowl.
2. In a separate bowl, beat together the pumpkin and eggs.
3. Add the dry ingredients to the wet and stir until smooth and well combined.
4. Grease a large skillet over medium-high heat.
5. Spoon the batter into the skillet using 2 to 3 tablespoons for each pancake.
6. Cook for 2 to 3 minutes until the underside is browned.
7. Carefully flip the pancakes and cook for another 2 minutes until browned underneath.
8. Transfer the cooked pancakes to a plate and repeat with the remaining batter.

Tomato Zucchini Omelet

Servings: 1

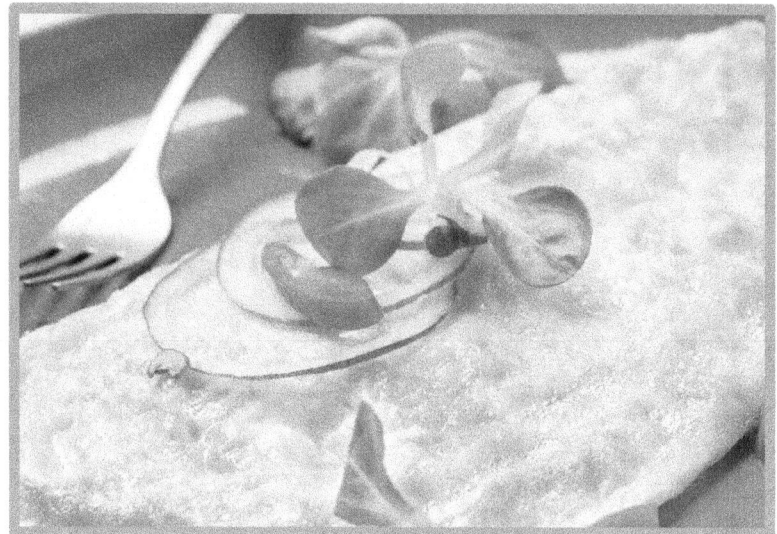

Ingredients:

- 2 large eggs
- Salt and pepper to taste
- 2 teaspoons olive oil
- 1 small tomato, chopped
- ¼ cup diced zucchini
- 1 green onion, sliced thin

Instructions:

1. Whisk together the eggs, salt and pepper in a small bowl and set aside.
2. Heat 1 teaspoon olive oil in a small skillet over medium-high heat.
3. Add the tomato and zucchini and cook for 3 minutes then remove to a bowl.
4. Reheat the skillet with the remaining 1 teaspoon olive oil.
5. Pour in the egg mixture and cook for 2 minutes, scraping down the sides of the pan.
6. When the egg is almost set, spoon the tomato and zucchini over half the omelet.
7. Fold the empty half of the omelet over the fillings and cook for another 1 to 2 minutes until set.
8. Slide the omelet onto a plate and garnish with green onion to serve.

Blueberry Coconut Pancakes

Servings: 4

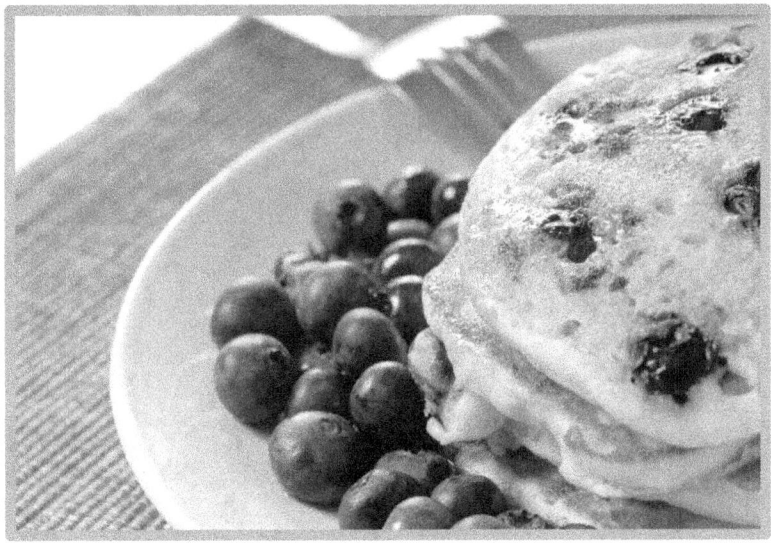

Ingredients:

- ½ cup coconut flour
- 1 cup unsweetened applesauce
- 5 large eggs, lightly beaten
- ¼ cup coconut oil
- 2 tablespoons unsweetened shredded coconut
- 2 tablespoons honey
- 1 teaspoon baking soda
- Pinch salt
- 1 cup fresh blueberries

Instructions:

1. Combine all of the ingredients except for the blueberries in a food processor and blend smooth.
2. Grease a large skillet and heat it over medium-high heat.
3. Spoon the batter into the skillet using 2 to 3 tablespoons per pancake.
4. Drop a few blueberries into the wet batter for each pancake and cook for 2 minutes.
5. Flip the pancakes when the underside is brown and cook for 1 minute more until browned underneath.
6. Transfer the pancakes to a plate to keep warm and repeat with the remaining batter.

Ham, Mushroom and Onion Frittata

Servings: 6

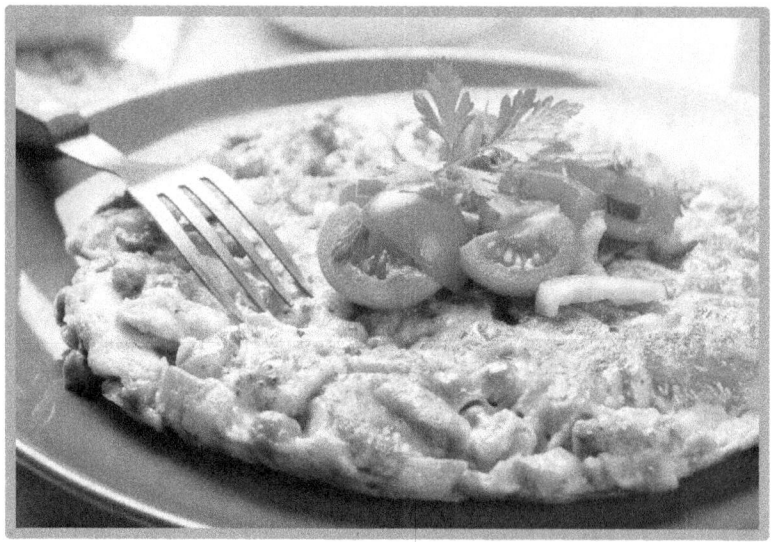

Ingredients:

- 1 tablespoon coconut oil
- 1 cup sliced mushrooms
- ½ cup diced onion
- 12 large eggs
- ¼ cup unsweetened almond milk
- Salt and pepper to taste

Instructions:

1. Heat the oil in a medium skillet over medium-high heat.
2. Add the mushrooms and onion and cook for 4 minutes, stirring often.
3. Whisk together the eggs, almond milk, salt and pepper and pour into the skillet.
4. Sprinkle with ham then cover and cook on medium-low heat for 15 minutes or so until the frittata is set.
5. Slide the frittata onto a plate and let sit for 3 to 4 minutes before cutting to serve.

Almond Flour Waffles

Servings: 2

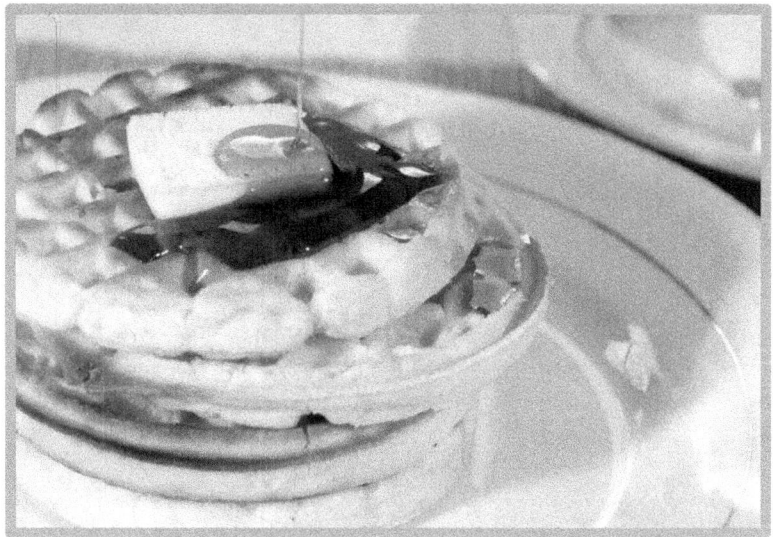

Ingredients:

- 2 large eggs, lightly beaten
- ¼ cup canned coconut milk
- 1 ½ cups almond flour
- ¼ cup unsweetened shredded coconut
- 1 tablespoon arrowroot powder
- 1 ½ tablespoons honey
- 1 teaspoon almond extract
- ½ teaspoon baking soda
- Pinch salt

Instructions:

1. Preheat your waffle iron to high heat.
2. Whisk together the eggs and coconut milk in a mixing bowl.
3. Add the almond flour and mix until smooth.
4. Beat in the coconut, arrowroot powder, baking soda, honey, almond extract and salt.
5. Blend smooth then spoon the batter into the waffle iron and cook as directed in the manufacturer's instructions.

Veggie Egg White Omelet

Servings: 1

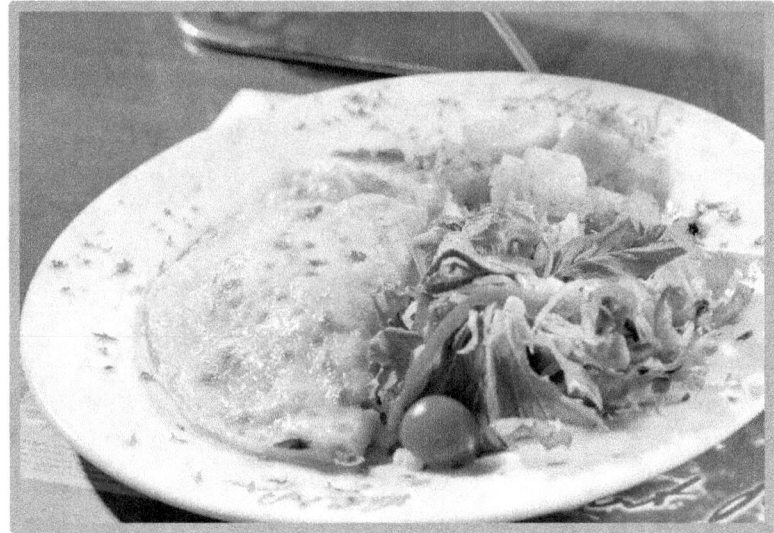

Ingredients:

- 4 large egg whites
- Salt and pepper to taste
- 2 teaspoons olive oil
- 1 small tomato, chopped
- 2 tablespoons diced zucchini
- 2 tablespoons diced onion
- 2 tablespoons diced red pepper
- 1 green onion, sliced thin

Instructions:

1. Whisk together the egg whites, salt and pepper in a small bowl and set aside.
2. Heat 1 teaspoon olive oil in a small skillet over medium-high heat.
3. Add the veggies and cook for 3 minutes then remove to a bowl.
4. Reheat the skillet with the remaining 1 teaspoon olive oil.
5. Pour in the egg mixture and cook for 2 minutes, scraping down the sides of the pan.
6. When the egg is almost set, spoon the veggies over half the omelet.

7. Fold the empty half of the omelet over the fillings and cook for another 1 to 2 minutes until set.
8. Slide the omelet onto a plate and garnish with green onion to serve.

Soup and Salad Recipes

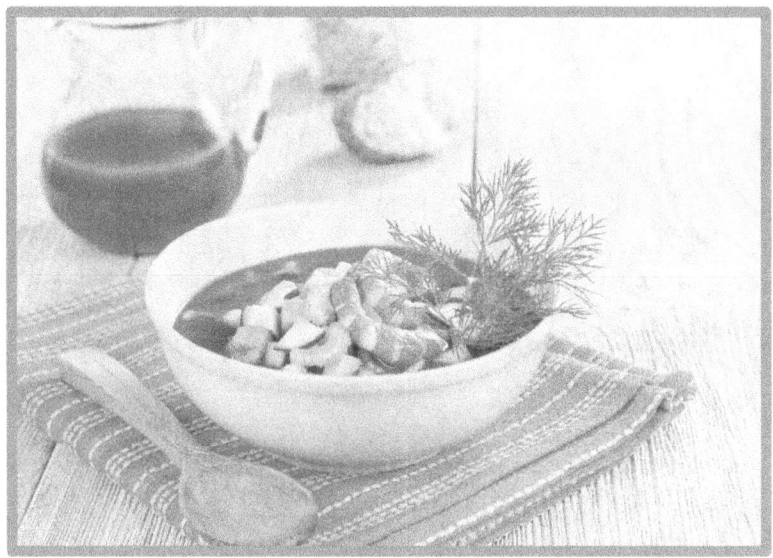

Recipes Included in this Section:

Roasted Tomato Onion Soup

Walnut Apple Kale Salad

Chicken Apple Salad

Creamy Beet Soup

Red Cabbage Carrot Salad

Cream of Spinach Soup

Vegetable Quinoa Salad

Roasted Tomato Onion Soup

Servings: 6

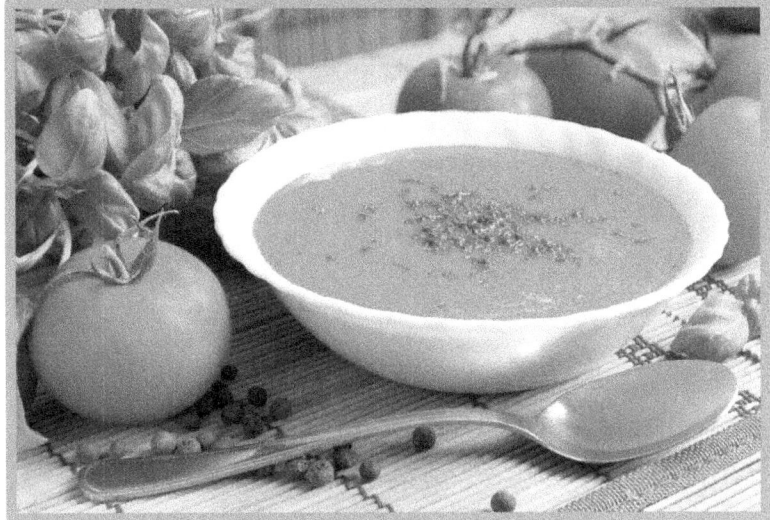

Ingredients:

- 2 ½ lbs. ripe Roma tomatoes, halved
- 1 large yellow onion, sliced
- 2 tablespoons olive oil
- Coarse salt
- 2 tablespoons coconut oil
- ½ cup diced carrots
- 1 (15 ounce) can diced tomatoes
- 4 cups vegetable broth
- ¼ cup fresh chopped basil

Instructions:

1. Preheat the oven to 400°F.
2. Line a rimmed baking sheet with foil and spread the tomatoes and onions on it.
3. Drizzle with olive oil and season liberally with salt and pepper.
4. Roast for 45 minutes, turning once halfway through.
5. Heat the coconut oil in a stockpot over medium heat.

6. Stir in the carrots and garlic and cook for 2 minutes.

7. Add the roasted vegetables along with the canned tomatoes, basil and vegetable broth.

8. Bring to a boil then reduce heat and simmer for 30 minutes.

9. Remove from heat and puree the soup using an immersion blender. Serve hot.

Walnut Apple Kale Salad

Servings: 2

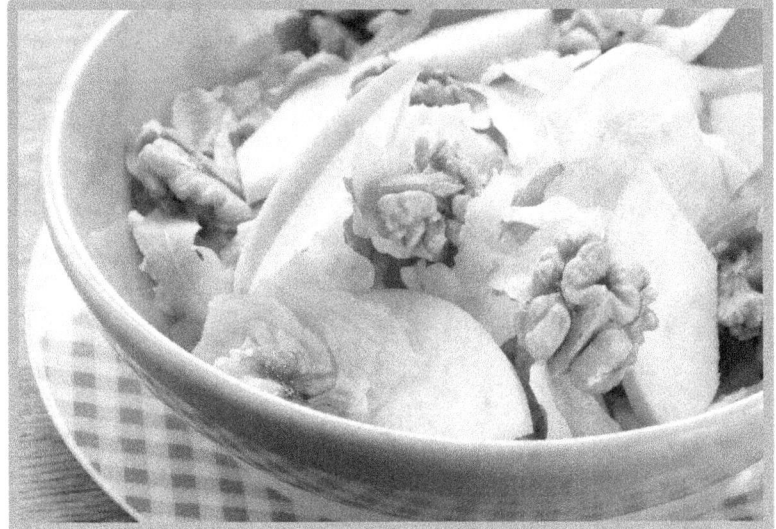

Ingredients:

- 4 cups chopped kale
- 1 medium green apple, sliced thin
- ¼ cup thinly sliced red onion
- ½ cup thinly sliced cucumber
- ¼ cup chopped walnuts
- 2 tablespoons olive oil
- 1 tablespoon white wine vinegar
- 1 tablespoon red wine vinegar
- ½ teaspoon honey
- Pinch salt

Instructions:

1. Combine the kale, apple, red onion and cucumber in a salad bowl.
2. Whisk together the remaining ingredients in a small bowl.
3. Toss the salad with the dressing and sprinkle with walnuts to serve.

Chicken Apple Salad

Servings: 4

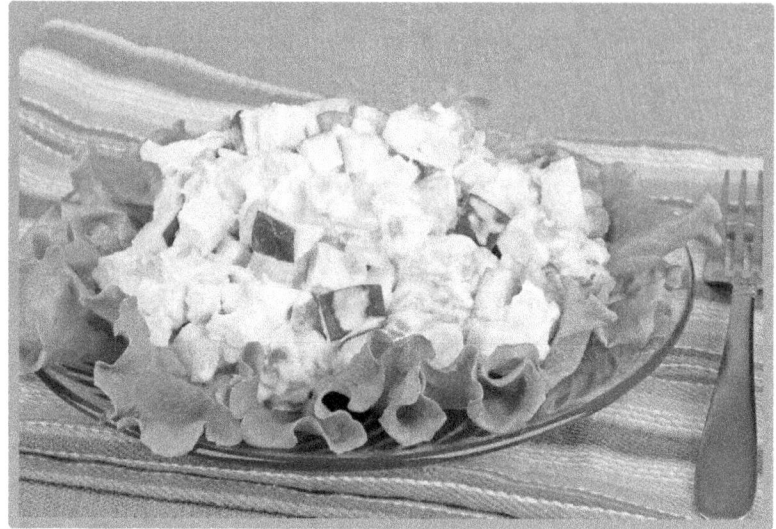

Ingredients:

- 1 lbs. cooked chicken breast, chopped
- 1 medium apple, peeled and chopped
- 1 cup diced celery
- ½ cup grapes, halved
- 1 ripe avocado, pitted and diced
- 1 cup mayonnaise
- 2 teaspoons lemon juice
- Salt and pepper to taste

Instructions:

1. Combine the chicken, celery, grapes, avocado and apple in a mixing bowl.
2. In a separate bowl, whisk together the mayonnaise, lemon juice, salt and pepper.
3. Toss the chicken mixture with the dressing to coat.
4. Chill until ready to serve.

Creamy Beet Soup

Servings: 4

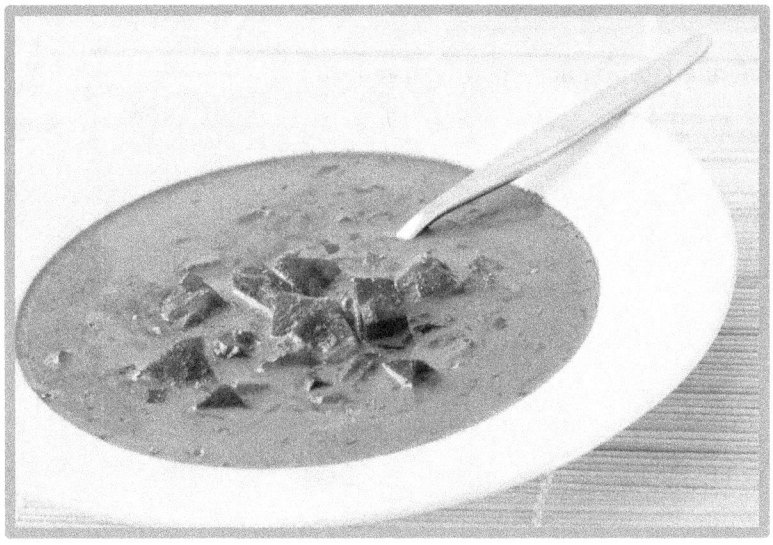

Ingredients:

- ½ lbs. red beets
- 1 tablespoon coconut oil
- 1 medium leek, rinsed and chopped
- 1 small yellow onion, chopped
- 1 medium stalk celery, chopped
- ¼ teaspoon ground ginger
- 1/8 teaspoon white pepper
- 2 cups water
- 1 bay leaf
- 1 teaspoon fresh thyme

Instructions:

1. Preheat the oven to 350°F.
2. Wrap the beets in foil and roast for 1 hour then let cool to room temperature.
3. Peel the beets then chop them into ¼-inch chunks.
4. Heat the oil in a large saucepan over medium-high heat.
5. Stir in the leek, onion and celery and cook for 10 minutes, stirring often.
6. Add the ginger and pepper and cook for 5 minutes more.
7. Stir in the water, bay leaf and thyme and bring to a boil.

8. Reduce heat and simmer for 25 minutes then remove the bay leaf and remove the pot from the heat.
9. Puree the soup using an immersion blender, setting aside 1 cup of soup to remain unblended.
10. Stir the unblended soup back in and serve hot.

Red Cabbage Carrot Salad

Servings: 6

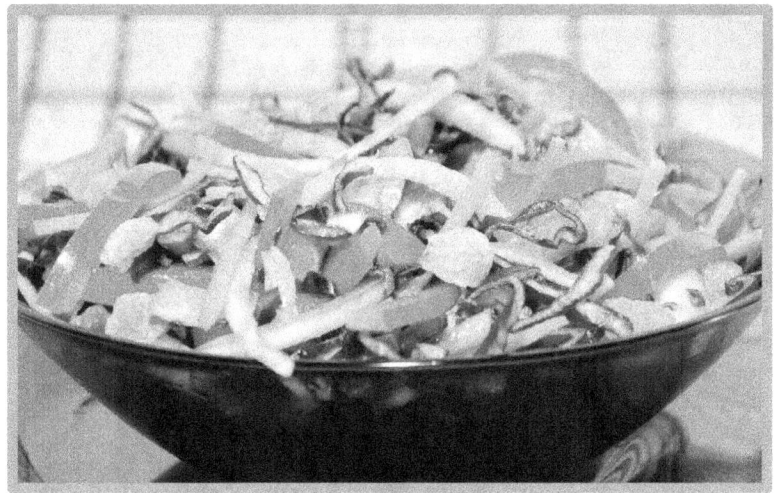

Ingredients:

- 4 cups shredded carrot
- 4 cups red cabbage, sliced thin
- 1 small red pepper, sliced thin
- ½ cup rice vinegar
- 1 tablespoon honey
- 1 teaspoon olive oil
- ½ teaspoon salt

Instructions:

1. Combine the vegetables in a salad bowl and mix well.
2. Whisk together the vinegar, honey, oil and salt in a small bowl then toss with the vegetables to coat.
3. Chill until ready to serve.

Cream of Spinach Soup

Servings: 6

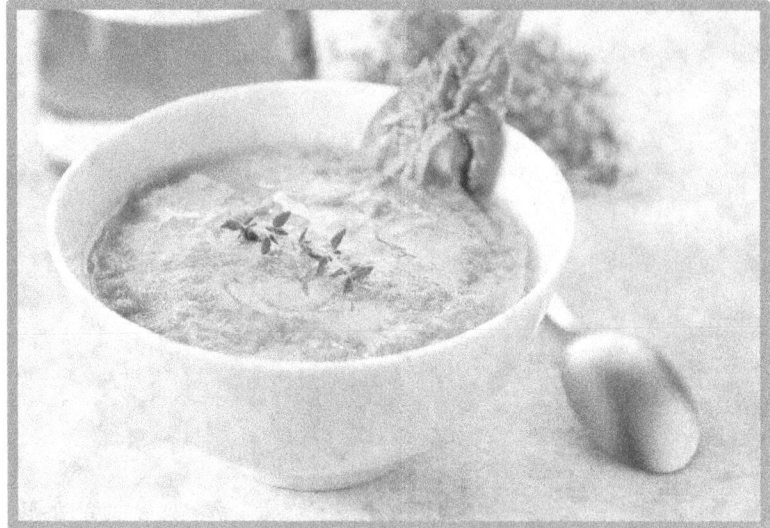

Ingredients:

- 2 tablespoons coconut oil
- 1 cup diced onion
- 1 lbs. potatoes, peeled and chopped
- 1 ½ cups chicken broth
- 1 ½ cups water
- 2 ½ cups fresh baby spinach, packed
- Salt and pepper to taste
- Chopped chives

Instructions:

1. Heat the oil in a large saucepan over medium heat.
2. Add the onion and cook for 3 minutes then stir in the potatoes, broth and water.
3. Bring the mixture to a boil then reduce heat and simmer for 20 minutes.
4. Stir in the spinach and cook for 2 minutes until wilted.
5. Remove from heat and puree the soup using an immersion blender.
6. Season with salt and pepper to taste and serve garnished with chopped chives.

Vegetable Quinoa Salad

Servings: 6

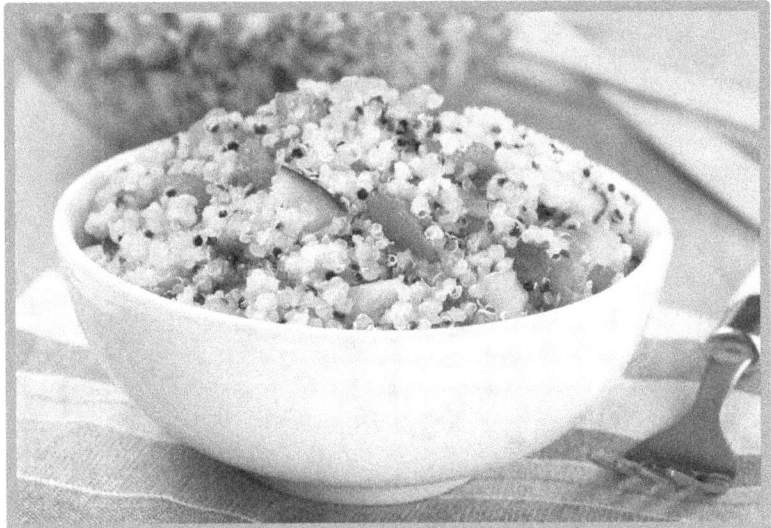

Ingredients:

- 1 ½ cups dry quinoa
- 3 cups water
- 1 teaspoon salt
- 2 tablespoons coconut oil
- 1 teaspoon minced garlic
- ½ cup diced onion
- 1 cup diced zucchini
- 1 small red pepper, diced
- 1 small yellow pepper, diced
- Salt and pepper to taste

Instructions:

1. Combine the quinoa, water and salt in a small saucepan and bring to a boil.
2. Reduce heat to low and simmer for 15 minutes.
3. Turn off the heat and let the quinoa stand for 5 minutes before fluffing with a fork.
4. Meanwhile, heat the oil in a medium skillet over medium-high heat.
5. Add the garlic and cook for 1 minute then stir in the onion, zucchini, red pepper and yellow pepper.
6. Cook for 6 to 8 minutes until tender then stir in the cooked quinoa.
7. Season with salt and pepper to taste and serve warm.

Main Entrée Recipes

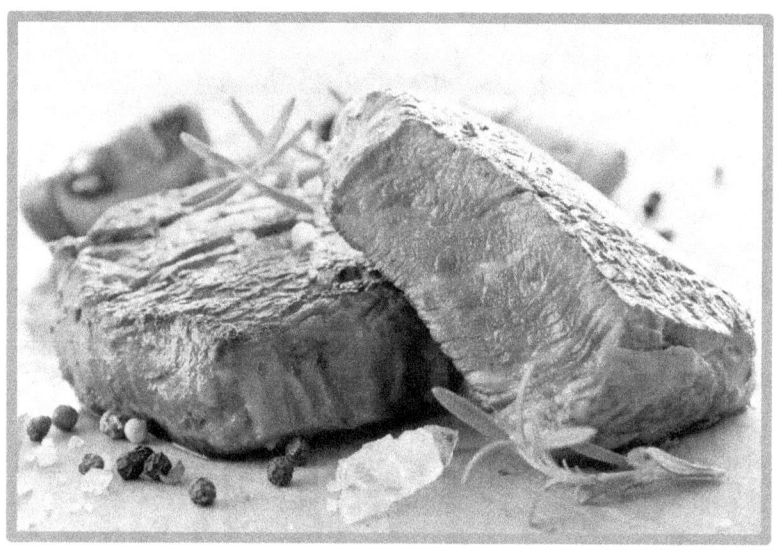

Recipes Included in this Section:

Cilantro Herbed Turkey Burgers

Lemon Garlic Pork Tenderloin

Chipotle Lime Shrimp

Spicy Turkey Chili

Slow-Cooker Pulled Pork

Oven-Roasted Beef Tenderloin

Ginger Broccoli Stir-Fry

Cilantro Herbed Turkey Burgers

Servings: 4

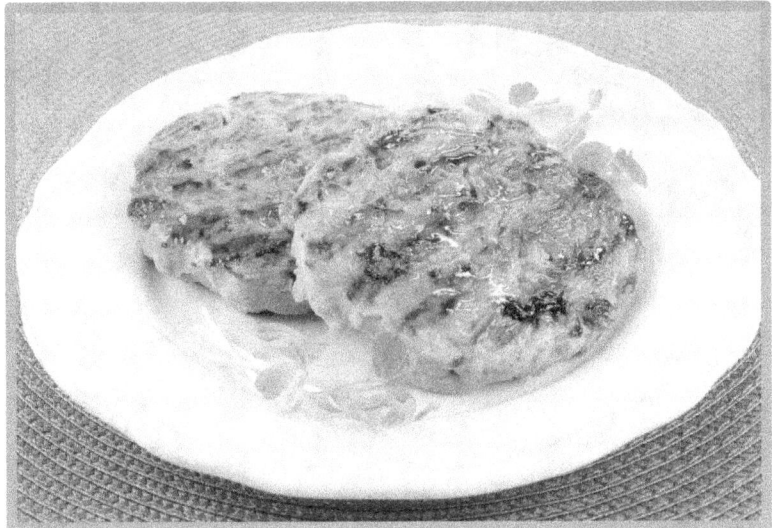

Ingredients:

- 1 lbs. lean ground turkey
- 1 tablespoon coconut flour
- 2 tablespoons fresh chopped cilantro
- 1 teaspoon dried oregano
- ¾ teaspoon salt
- ¼ teaspoon black pepper

Instructions:

1. Preheat the broiler in your oven to high heat.
2. Combine all of the ingredients in a large mixing bowl and stir well.
3. Shape the mixture into patties by hand and pat them to about ½-inch thick.
4. Place the patties on a broiler pan and broil for 4 to 5 minutes on each side until cooked through.
5. Serve hot with your favorite burger toppings.

Lemon Garlic Pork Tenderloin

Servings: 8

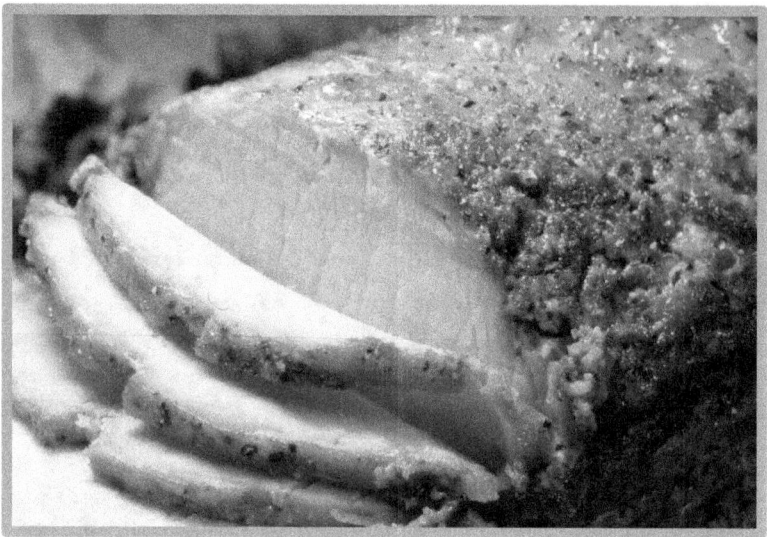

Ingredients:

- 1 (2 ½ lbs.) boneless pork tenderloin
- Salt and pepper to taste
- 1 tablespoon minced garlic
- 2 teaspoons dried rosemary
- 2 teaspoon fresh lemon zest

Instructions:

1. Preheat the oven to 400°F and line a roasting pan with foil.
2. Combine the garlic, rosemary and lemon zest in a small bowl.
3. Season the pork with salt and pepper to taste then rub the garlic lemon mixture into the pork on all sides.
4. Place the roast, fat-side-down, in the roasting pan.
5. Roast for 30 minutes then turn it right side up and roast for another 25 minutes or so until the internal temperature reaches 155°F.
6. Remove the roast to a cutting board and let rest for 10 minutes before slicing to serve.

Chipotle Lime Shrimp

Servings: 4

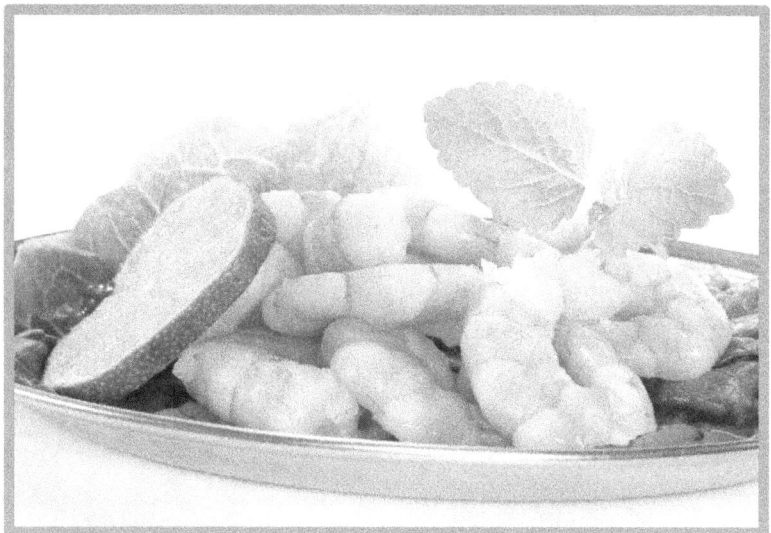

Ingredients:

- 1 ½ lbs. uncooked shrimp, peeled and deveined
- ¼ cup olive oil
- 2 tablespoons fresh lime juice
- 1 teaspoon fresh lime zest
- 1 teaspoon minced garlic
- 1 teaspoon chipotle chili powder
- ½ teaspoon salt
- Lime wedges

Instructions:

1. Rinse the shrimp well in cool water then pat dry with paper towels.
2. Whisk together the remaining ingredients in a small bowl.
3. Place the shrimp in a plastic freezer bag and pour in the marinade.
4. Shake well to coat then chill in the refrigerator for 30 minutes.
5. Preheat a stove-top grill pan over medium high heat.
6. Arrange the shrimp on the grill pan in a single layer.

7. Cook for 1 to 2 minutes then turn the shrimp and cook for another 1 to 2 minutes until bright pink and just cooked through.

8. Serve the shrimp hot with lime wedges.

Spicy Turkey Chili

Servings: 6

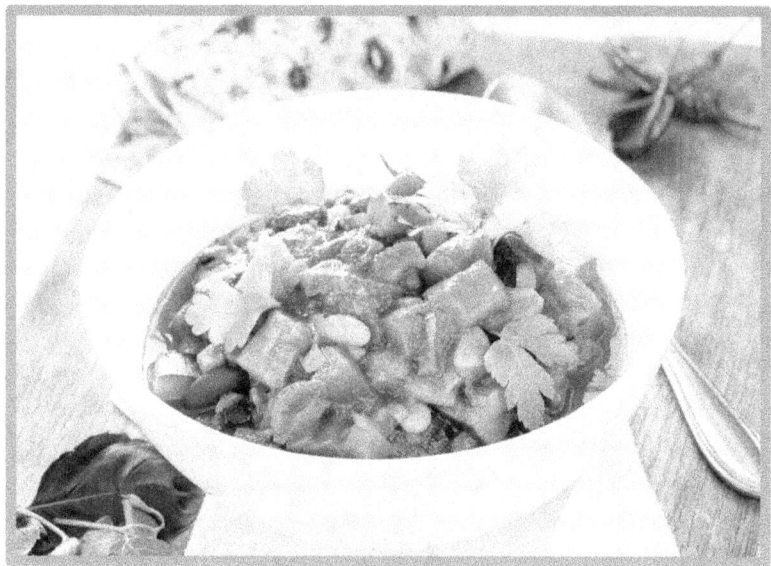

Ingredients:

- 2 tablespoons olive oil

- 1 large yellow onion, diced

- 1 red pepper, diced

- 1 green pepper, diced

- 1 tablespoon chili powder

- 1 tablespoon chipotle chili powder

- 1 jalapeno pepper, seeded and minced

- Salt to taste

- 1 (28-ounce) can whole tomatoes, with juice

- 1 (14.5 ounce) can black beans, rinsed and drained

- ½ cup water

- 1 lbs. lean ground turkey

Instructions:

1. Heat the oil in a stockpot over medium heat.

2. Add the onion and peppers and cook for 10 minutes until they are tender and browned.

3. Stir in the chili powder, chipotle chili powder and jalapeno and cook for 1 minute.

4. Add the tomatoes, beans and water then season with salt to taste.

5. Stir in the ground turkey and simmer for 20 minutes or so until the turkey is cooked through and the beans are tender.

6. Let stand for 5 minutes before serving.

Slow-Cooker Pulled Pork

Servings: 6

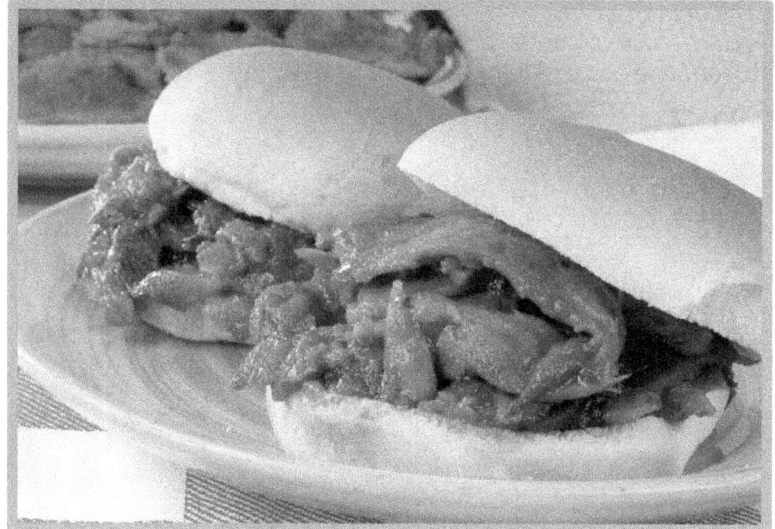

Ingredients:

- 2 large yellow onions, sliced
- 1 tablespoon minced garlic
- 1 cup chicken broth
- 1 tablespoon chili powder
- 1 tablespoon coarse salt
- 1 teaspoon ground cumin
- ½ teaspoon ground cinnamon
- 1 (4 ½ to 5 lbs.) boneless pork shoulder

Instructions:

1. Spread the onions and garlic in the bottom of a slow cooker and pour in the chicken broth.
2. Whisk together the chili powder, salt, cumin and cinnamon in a small bowl.
3. Rub the spice mixture into the pork and place it in the slow cooker over the onions.
4. Cover and cook on high for 6 to 8 hours or on low for 8 to 10 hours until tender.

5. Remove the pork to a cutting board and strain the remaining contents of the slow cooker into a bowl – reserve the liquid.

6. Shred the pork using two forks and return it to the slow cooker.

7. Skim the fat from the reserved liquid and stir in about ¼ cup of it at a time until the pork is moist.

8. Season with salt and pepper to taste then serve hot.

Oven-Roasted Beef Tenderloin

Servings: 8

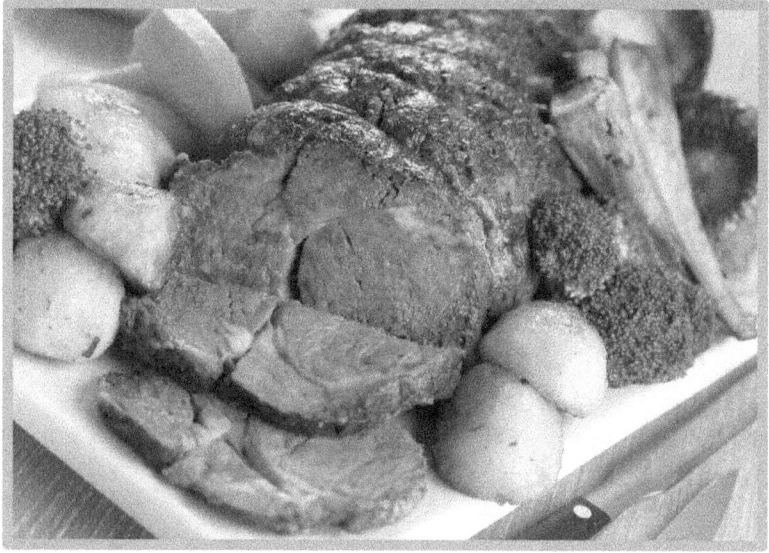

Ingredients:

- 1 (2-3 pound) boneless beef tenderloin
- Salt and pepper to taste
- 2 tablespoons fresh chopped rosemary
- 2 teaspoons minced garlic
- 1 teaspoon dried thyme
- 1 large yellow onion, sliced
- 1 ½ lbs. red potatoes, quartered
- 1 lbs. sliced carrots
- ¼ cup beef broth

Instructions:

1. Preheat the oven to 400°F.
2. Season the beef liberally with salt and pepper to taste.
3. Sprinkle with rosemary, garlic and thyme then set aside.
4. Heat the oil in a large skillet over medium-high heat.

5. Add the beef tenderloin and cook for 2 to 3 minutes on each side until evenly browned, about 10 minutes total.

6. Combine the potatoes, carrots and onions in a large roasting pan and place the tenderloin on top.

7. Drizzle the beef broth over the vegetables.

8. Roast the beef for 20 to 25 minutes until its internal temperature reaches at least 130°F.

9. Transfer the beef to a cutting board and let rest, covered with foil, for 10 minutes before carving to serve.

10. Serve the beef hot with the roasted vegetables.

Ginger Broccoli Stir-Fry

Servings: 6

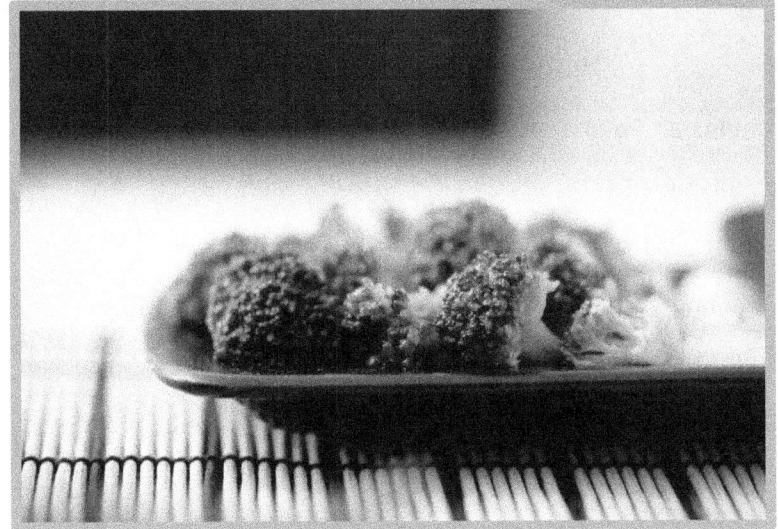

Ingredients:

- 3 tablespoons plus 1 teaspoon olive oil, divided
- 3 cups broccoli florets, chopped
- 1 cup chopped carrots
- 1 large yellow onion, chopped
- ½ medium red pepper, chopped
- ½ medium green pepper, chopped
- 1 tablespoon fresh minced ginger
- 1 tablespoon fresh minced garlic
- ¼ cup coconut aminos
- 1 tablespoon sesame oil
- 1 teaspoon arrowroot powder
- 1 cup shredded cabbage

Instructions:

1. Heat 2 tablespoons of olive oil in a large skillet over medium-high heat.
2. Add the broccoli and toss to coat with oil.

3. Sauté the broccoli for 5 to 7 minutes until bright green and crisp.

4. Transfer the broccoli to a bowl to keep warm and reheat the skillet with another 1 tablespoon olive oil.

5. Add the carrots and cook for 3 minutes, tossing often.

6. Stir in the onions and bell peppers and cook for 4 to 5 minutes, stirring often, until the onions are translucent.

7. Transfer all of the vegetables to the bowl with the broccoli.

8. Add the remaining 1 teaspoon olive oil to the skillet and stir in the ginger and garlic.

9. Cook for 1 minute until fragrant and hot.

10. Whisk together the remaining ingredients aside from the cabbage and pour into the skillet.

11. Cook for 1 to 2 minutes until hot and bubbling then stir in the vegetables.

12. Add the cabbage and toss everything to coat.

13. Cook for 1 to 2 minutes until heated through and the cabbage is just softened.

14. Serve hot over a bed of steamed rice.

Dessert Recipes

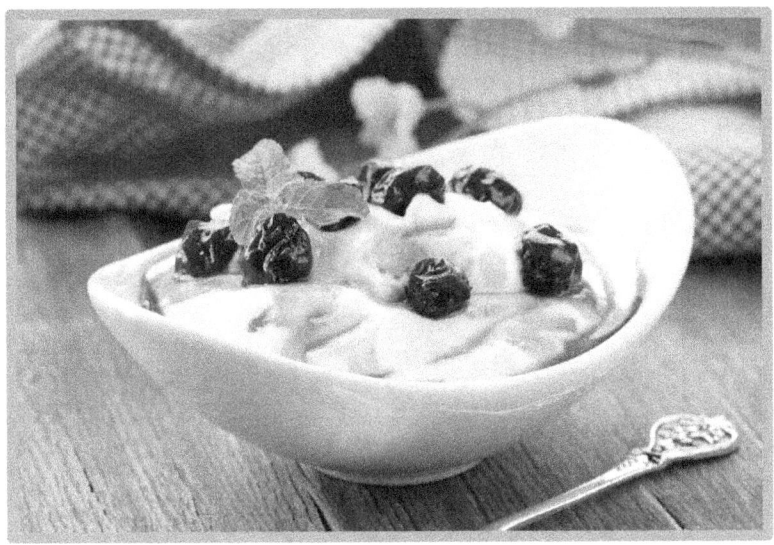

Recipes Included in this Section:

Lemon Pudding

Blueberry Crumble

Maple Pecan Cookies

Almond Flour Cupcakes

Strawberry Lime Sorbet

Baked Apples with Walnuts

Chocolate Coconut Cupcakes

Lemon Pudding

Servings: 4

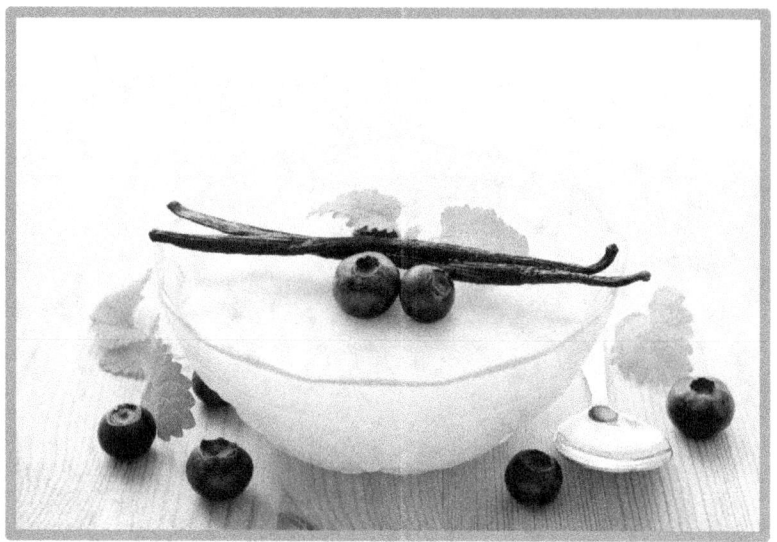

Ingredients:

- 1 (14.5 ounce) can full-fat coconut milk
- Juice from 1 lemon
- Zest from 1 lemon
- ¾ teaspoon vanilla extract
- 2 ½ tablespoons honey
- 1 teaspoon powdered gelatin
- 3 large egg yolks

Instructions:

1. Combine the coconut milk, lemon juice, lemon zest, vanilla extract, honey and gelatin in a medium saucepan.
2. Heat the saucepan over medium heat and whisk in the egg yolks.
3. Stir for 5 to 7 minutes until heated and bubbling – do not boil.
4. Remove from heat and spoon into dessert cups.
5. Chill until ready to serve – at least 4 hours.

Blueberry Crumble

Servings: 4

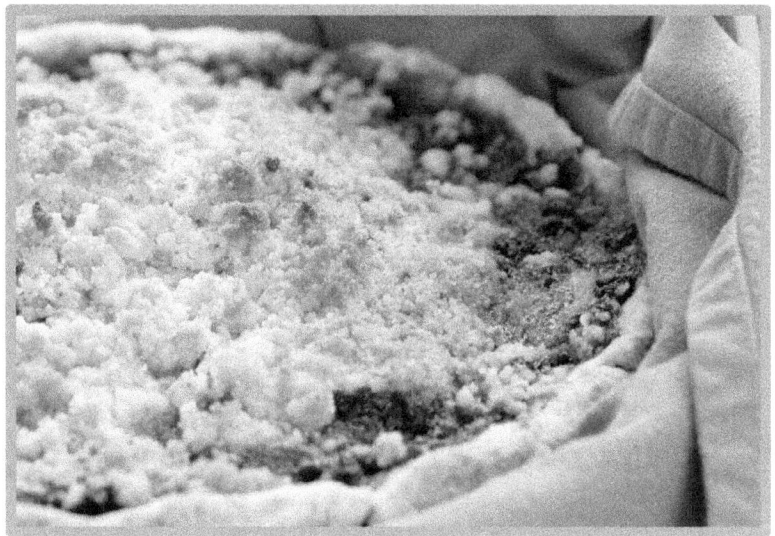

Ingredients:

- 4 cups fresh blueberries
- 1 cup almond flour
- ¼ cup coconut oil
- 1 teaspoon vanilla extract
- 2 tablespoons honey

Instructions:

1. Preheat the oven to 375°F and grease an 8x8-inch glass baking dish.
2. Combine the almond flour, coconut oil and vanilla extract in a bowl until it forms a crumbly mixture.
3. Place the blueberries in the baking dish and sprinkle the crumble over top.
4. Bake for 20 minutes then drizzle with honey to serve.

Maple Pecan Cookies

Servings: 24

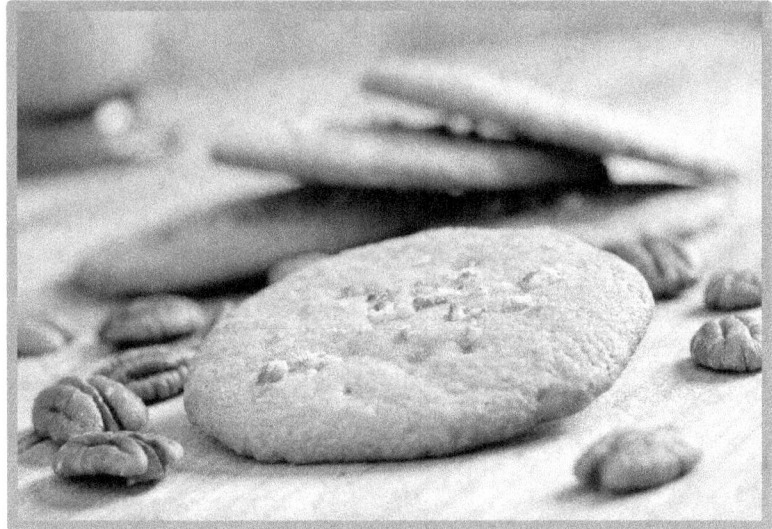

Ingredients:

- 2 ½ cups almond flour
- ¼ teaspoon baking soda
- ¼ teaspoon salt
- 2/3 cup coconut oil, melted
- ½ cup maple syrup
- 2 teaspoons vanilla extract
- 1 cup chopped pecans

Instructions:

1. Preheat the oven to 350°F and line a baking sheet with parchment paper.
2. Combine the almond flour, baking soda and salt in a mixing bowl.
3. In a separate bowl, beat together the coconut oil, maple syrup and vanilla extract.
4. Mix the dry ingredients into the wet until well combined.
5. Fold in the chopped pecans then drop the batter onto the prepared cooking sheet in 1-inch balls.
6. Bake for 7 to 10 minutes until lightly browned.

7. Cool on a wire cooling rack before serving.

Almond Flour Cupcakes

Servings: 12

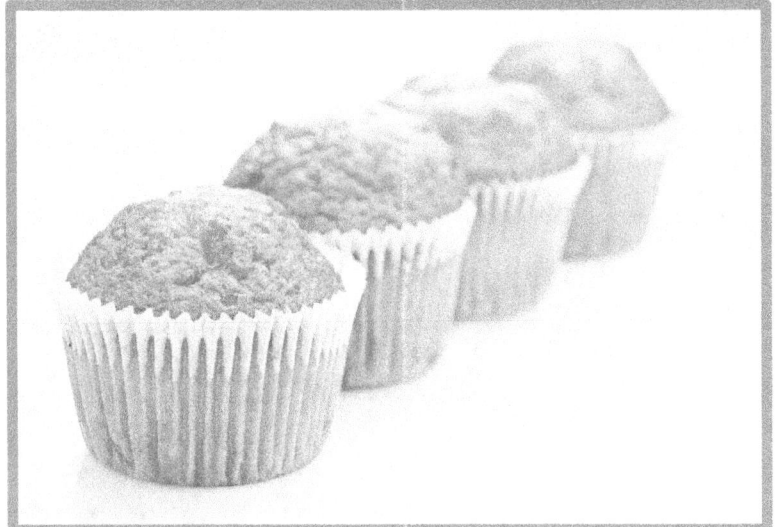

Ingredients:

- ½ cup sifted coconut flour
- ¼ teaspoon baking soda
- ¼ teaspoon salt
- 6 large eggs, lightly beaten
- ½ cup coconut oil, melted
- ½ cup honey
- 2 teaspoons vanilla extract

Instructions:

1. Preheat the oven to 350°F and line a regular muffin pan with paper liners.
2. Combine the coconut flour, baking soda and salt in a mixing bowl.
3. In a separate bowl, whisk together the eggs, coconut oil, honey and vanilla extract.
4. Add the wet ingredients to the dry and whisk until smooth and well combined.
5. Spoon the batter into the prepared pan, filling each cup about 2/3 full.
6. Bake for 18 to 20 minutes until a knife inserted in the center comes out clean.
7. Cool the cupcakes on a wire rack.

Strawberry Lime Sorbet

Servings: 4

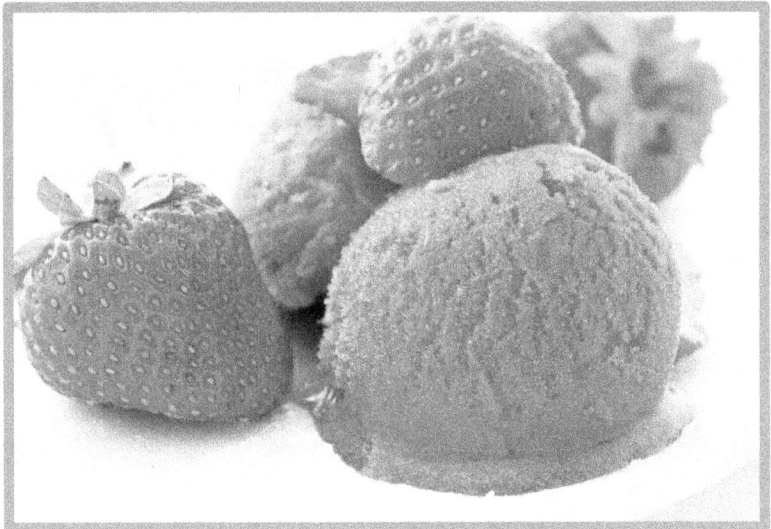

Ingredients:

- 10 ounces frozen strawberries
- 1 ½ cups water
- ½ cup fresh lime juice
- ¼ cup honey

Instructions:

1. Combine the strawberries, water and lime juice in a blender.
2. Blend on high speed until smooth and combined.
3. Pour the mixture into an ice cream maker and freeze according to the manufacturer's instructions.

Baked Apples with Walnuts

Servings: 4

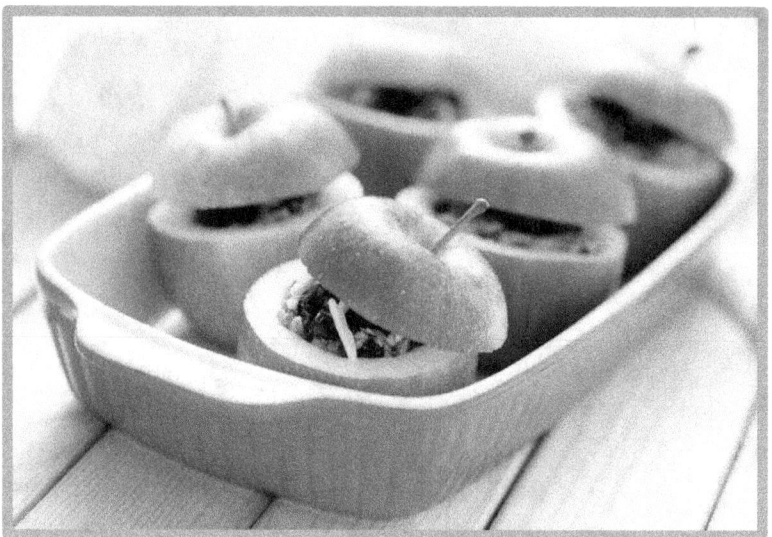

Ingredients:

- 4 ripe apples
- ½ cup shredded unsweetened coconut
- ¼ cup finely chopped walnuts
- 1 teaspoon ground cinnamon
- ½ teaspoon ground nutmeg

Instructions:

1. Preheat the oven to 350°F.
2. Cut the tops off the apples and carefully scoop out the core.
3. Arrange the apples in a glass baking dish.
4. Stir together the coconut, walnuts, cinnamon and nutmeg in a small bowl then spoon the mixture into the apples.
5. Place the tops back on the apples and bake for 25 to 30 minutes until tender.

Chocolate Coconut Cupcakes

Servings: 12

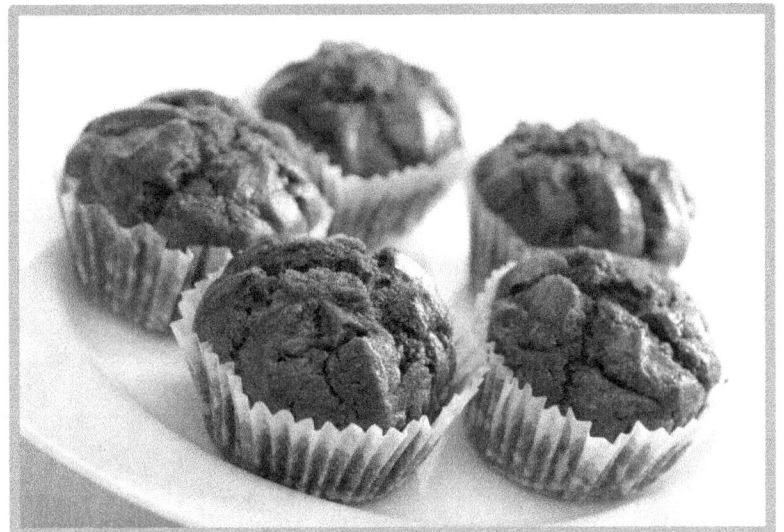

Ingredients:

- ¼ cup coconut flour
- ¼ cup unsweetened cocoa powder
- ½ cup unsweetened shredded coconut
- 3 large eggs
- ½ cup raw honey
- ¼ cup coconut oil, melted
- 1 teaspoon vanilla extract
- ½ teaspoon baking soda
- Pinch salt

Instructions:

1. Preheat the oven to 375°F and line a regular muffin pan with paper liners.
2. Combine the coconut flour, cocoa powder, baking soda and salt in a mixing bowl.
3. In a separate bowl, whisk together the eggs, honey, coconut oil and vanilla extract.
4. Add the dry ingredients to the wet and blend smooth then fold in the coconut.
5. Spoon the batter into the prepared pan, filling the cups about 2/3 full.

6. Bake for 20 to 22 minutes until a knife inserted in the center comes out clean.

Chapter Four: 7-Day Detox Plan

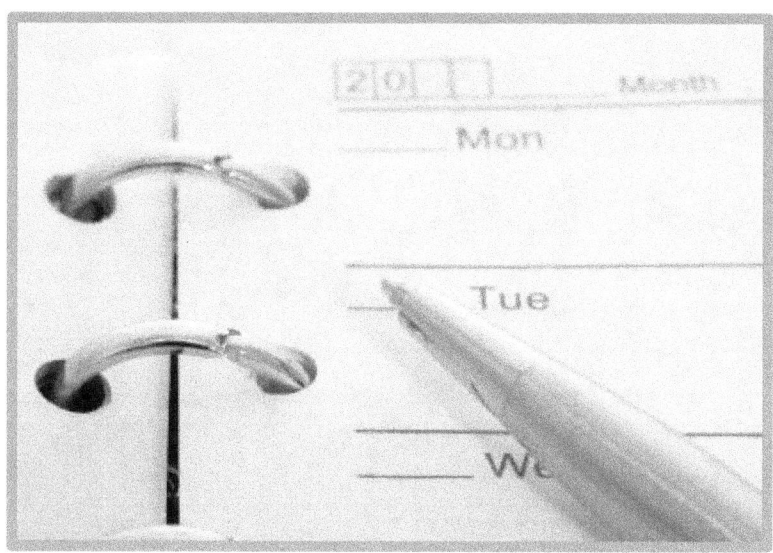

Use the recipes in this book to get started on your 7-day liver detox plan. Below you will find a sample meal plan to use as a suggestion when planning your detox.

Day	**Breakfast**	**Lunch**	**Dinner**	**Dessert**
1	Banana Nut Muffins	Roasted Tomato Onion Soup	Cilantro Herbed Turkey Burgers	Lemon Pudding
2	Pumpkin Spice Pancakes	Walnut Apple Kale Salad	Lemon Garlic Pork Tenderloin	Blueberry Crumble
3	Tomato Zucchini Omelet	Chicken Apple Salad	Chipotle Lime Shrimp	Maple Pecan Cookies
4	Blueberry Coconut Pancakes	Creamy Beet Soup	Spicy Turkey Chili	Almond Flour Cupcakes
5	Ham, Mushroom and Onion Frittata	Red Cabbage Carrot Salad	Slow-Cooker Pulled Pork	Strawberry Lime Sorbet
6	Almond Flour Waffles	Cream of Spinach Soup	Oven-Roasted Beef Tenderloin	Baked Apples with Walnuts
7	Veggie Egg White Omelet	Vegetable Quinoa Salad	Ginger Broccoli Stir-Fry	Chocolate Coconut Cupcakes

Conclusion

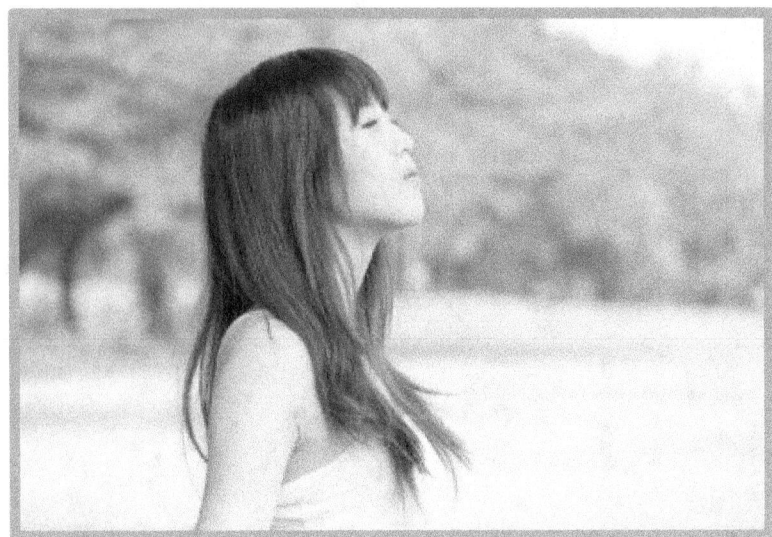

After reading this book you should understand the basics of what a detox is and why it is good for your body. More specifically, you should have learned why it is important to detox and take care of your liver. You also received valuable tips for planning and implementing your own 7-day liver detox using the collection of delicious detoxifying recipes provided.

Thanks for reading and good luck with your detox!

www.ingramcontent.com/pod-product-compliance
Lightning Source LLC
Chambersburg PA
CBHW081751280526
45789CB00008B/2813